CHAPTER 1

The Importance of Personal Hygiene: A Gateway to Health and Well-being

Personal hygiene is more than just looking and smelling good; it's a fundamental aspect of maintaining overall health and well-being. From preventing the spread of infectious diseases to boosting self-confidence, practicing good hygiene habits plays a crucial role in our daily lives. In this blog, we'll explore the importance of personal hygiene and its far-reaching impact on our physical, mental, and social health.

Understanding Personal Hygiene

Personal hygiene encompasses a range of practices aimed at promoting cleanliness and preventing the spread of germs and bacteria. These practices include:

1. **Regular Handwashing:** Washing hands with soap and water is one of the most effective ways to prevent the spread of infectious diseases, such as colds, flu, and gastrointestinal illnesses.

2. **Showering and Bathing:** Regular bathing helps to remove dirt, sweat, and bacteria from the skin, reducing the risk of skin infections and unpleasant body odors.

3. **Oral Hygiene:** Brushing and flossing teeth regularly, along with routine dental check-ups, are essential for maintaining oral health and preventing tooth decay, gum disease, and bad breath.

4. **Proper Clothing and Footwear:** Wearing clean clothes and changing socks regularly helps to prevent the buildup of sweat and bacteria, reducing the risk of skin infections and foot odor.

5. **Healthy Diet and Hydration:** Consuming a balanced diet rich in fruits, vegetables, and whole grains, along with staying

hydrated, supports overall health and can have a positive impact on skin, hair, and nail health.

The Impact on Physical Health

Practicing good personal hygiene habits can have a profound impact on physical health by reducing the risk of illness and infection. For example:

Preventing Disease Transmission: Proper handwashing can significantly reduce the transmission of infectious diseases, such as the common cold, flu, and foodborne illnesses.

Reducing Skin Infections: Regular bathing and skincare help to remove bacteria and prevent skin infections, such as acne, athlete's foot, and dermatitis.

Maintaining Oral Health: Good oral hygiene habits, including brushing, flossing, and routine dental check-ups, are essential for preventing tooth decay, gum disease, and other oral health issues.

Preventing Respiratory Infections: Covering the mouth and nose when coughing or sneezing, along with proper disposal of tissues, can help prevent the spread of respiratory infections, such as the flu and COVID-19.

The Psychological and Social Benefits

In addition to its physical benefits, practicing good personal hygiene can have positive effects on mental and social well-being:

Boosting Self-Confidence: Feeling clean and well-groomed can boost self-confidence and self-esteem, leading to improved mental well-being and a more positive self-image.

Enhancing Social Relationships: Maintaining good personal hygiene is important for social interactions, as it helps to prevent body odor and bad breath, making people more comfortable to be around.

Improving Mood: Engaging in regular hygiene practices, such as bathing and grooming, can promote relaxation and reduce stress, leading to improved mood and overall emotional well-being.

Cultural and Societal Norms

The importance of personal hygiene is influenced by cultural and societal norms, which vary widely across different cultures and communities. While some hygiene practices may be universal, others may be specific to certain cultural traditions or religious beliefs. Regardless of cultural differences, maintaining good personal hygiene is universally recognized as essential for promoting health and well-being.

Conclusion

In conclusion, personal hygiene is a cornerstone of good health and well-being. By adopting simple hygiene practices such as handwashing, bathing, and oral care, individuals can protect themselves and others from illness and infection, boost their self-confidence, and enhance their overall quality of life. It's essential to educate ourselves and others about the importance of personal hygiene and to incorporate these practices into our daily routines for a healthier, happier future.

Chapter 2

Daily Skincare Routine: Unveiling the Secrets to Healthy, Glowing Skin

In our fast-paced lives, taking care of our skin can often be neglected amidst the chaos of daily routines. However, investing time and effort into a daily skincare routine is essential for maintaining healthy, radiant skin. This chapter serves as your comprehensive guide to understanding the fundamentals of skincare, from cleansing and moisturizing to safeguarding against the sun's harmful rays.

Cleansing: The First Step to Clean, Clear Skin

The cornerstone of any skincare routine is cleansing. Cleansing helps to remove dirt, oil, makeup, and impurities that accumulate on the skin throughout the day. It's essential to choose a gentle cleanser suitable for your skin type – whether it's oily, dry, combination, or sensitive.

For oily or acne-prone skin, opt for a foaming or gel-based cleanser that helps to unclog pores and control excess oil production. Those with dry or sensitive skin should choose a creamy or hydrating cleanser that cleanses without stripping away natural oils.

When cleansing the skin, it's important to use lukewarm water and gentle, circular motions to avoid irritation. Be sure to cleanse both morning and night to maintain a clean canvas for the rest of your skincare routine.

How Often Should You Cleanse:

The frequency of cleansing depends on your skin type and lifestyle factors. As a general rule of thumb, it's recommended to cleanse your face twice daily – once in the morning and once at night – to remove dirt, oil, and impurities. However, if you have oily or acne-prone skin, you may benefit from cleansing more frequently, especially after sweating or exercising.

Types of Cleansers:

Not all cleansers are created equal, and choosing the right one for your skin type is essential for achieving optimal results. Here's a breakdown of the different types of cleansers and their ideal uses:

1. Gel Cleansers: Ideal for oily and acne-prone skin, gel cleansers are lightweight and effective at removing excess oil and impurities without stripping the skin of its natural moisture. Look for ingredients like salicylic acid or tea tree oil to help combat acne and blemishes.

2. Cream Cleansers: Best suited for dry or sensitive skin types, cream cleansers are gentle and hydrating, leaving the skin feeling soft and nourished. They work by effectively removing dirt and makeup while maintaining the skin's moisture barrier. Ingredients like glycerine and hyaluronic acid are beneficial for maintaining hydration.

3. Foam Cleansers: Foam cleansers are excellent for combination or normal skin types, providing a thorough

cleanse without overdrying the skin. They lather up to remove dirt, oil, and makeup, leaving the skin feeling refreshed and balanced. Look for gentle, non-stripping formulas to avoid disrupting the skin's natural pH balance.

4. Micellar Water: Micellar water is a versatile cleanser suitable for all skin types, including sensitive skin. It contains micelles, tiny oil molecules that attract and lift away dirt, oil, and makeup without the need for rinsing. Simply soak a cotton pad with micellar water and gently swipe it across the face to cleanse and refresh the skin.

5. Oil Cleansers: Contrary to popular belief, oil cleansers are suitable for all skin types, including oily and acne-prone skin. They work on the principle of "like dissolves like," effectively removing excess oil, sunscreen, and makeup without stripping the skin. Oil cleansers are especially beneficial for removing stubborn waterproof makeup and sunscreen.

Now that we've covered the basics let's dive into a step-by-step cleansing routine for healthy, radiant skin:

1. Start by wetting your face with lukewarm water to help open up the pores and prepare the skin for cleansing.
2. Dispense a small amount of cleanser onto your fingertips and gently massage it onto your skin in circular motions, focusing on areas with excess oil, dirt, or makeup.
3. Rinse thoroughly with lukewarm water, making sure to remove all traces of cleanser from the skin.
4. Pat your skin dry with a clean towel, being careful not to rub or tug on the delicate skin.

5. Follow up with your favourite toner, serum, moisturizer, and sunscreen to lock in hydration and protect the skin from environmental damage.

Conclusion:

A daily cleansing routine is the foundation of healthy, radiant skin. By choosing the right cleanser for your skin type and following a consistent skincare regimen, you can effectively remove dirt, oil, makeup, and impurities, leaving your skin refreshed, balanced, and glowing. So, why wait? Start your journey towards healthier skin today!

Chapter 3

Moisturizing: Nourishing Your Skin for Optimal Hydration

After cleansing, the next step in your skincare routine should be moisturizing. Moisturizers help to hydrate the skin, replenish moisture levels, and create a protective barrier to lock in hydration. Regardless of your skin type, moisturizing is essential for maintaining a healthy skin barrier and preventing issues such as dryness, flakiness, and irritation.

When choosing a moisturizer, consider your skin type and any specific concerns you may have. For oily or acne-prone skin, opt for a lightweight, oil-free moisturizer that won't clog pores. Dry skin types may benefit from a richer, cream-based moisturizer that provides intense hydration.

In addition to choosing the right moisturizer, it's important to apply it correctly. After cleansing, gently pat your skin dry with a clean towel and then apply a pea-sized amount of moisturizer to your face and neck. Massage the moisturizer into your skin using upward, circular motions, ensuring thorough coverage.Unlocking the Secrets of Skin Moisturization: Your Ultimate Guide to Hydrated, Glowing Skin

In the quest for radiant, supple skin, moisturization reigns supreme. Yet, amidst the sea of moisturizers and skincare advice, finding the perfect formula and routine tailored to your skin's needs can feel like a daunting task. Fear not! In this comprehensive guide, we'll delve into the world of moisturization, from understanding different skin types and moisturizer formulations to mastering application techniques for maximum efficacy. By the end, you'll be equipped with the knowledge to achieve your skin's ultimate hydration goals.

Understanding Your Skin: The Key to Effective Moisturization

Before delving into the intricacies of moisturization, it's crucial to understand your skin type. Our skin falls into several categories, each with its unique characteristics and needs:

1. **Dry Skin:** Dry skin tends to feel tight, rough, and may exhibit flakiness or even cracks. It lacks natural oils (sebum) and struggles to retain moisture, leading to dehydration.

2. **Oily Skin:** Oily skin is characterized by excessive sebum production, resulting in a shiny or greasy appearance, enlarged pores, and a predisposition to acne or breakouts.

3. **Combination Skin:** Combination skin features a mix of oily and dry areas, with the T-zone (forehead, nose, and chin) typically being oilier while the cheeks remain drier.

4. **Normal Skin:** Lucky individuals with normal skin experience a balanced complexion, neither too oily nor too dry, with minimal sensitivity and few blemishes.

5. **Sensitive Skin:** Sensitive skin is prone to irritation, redness, and inflammation, reacting adversely to harsh ingredients or environmental triggers.

Understanding your skin type is essential for selecting the right moisturizer and formulating an effective skincare routine.

Types of Moisturizers: Choosing the Right Formula

Now that we've decoded your skin type, let's explore the various types of moisturizers available:

1. **Creams:** Creams are thicker in consistency and provide intense hydration, making them ideal for dry or mature skin types. They often contain occlusive ingredients like petrolatum or shea butter, which lock in moisture and create a protective barrier against environmental aggressors.

2. **Lotions:** Lotions are lighter than creams and suitable for normal to combination skin types. They offer hydration without feeling heavy or greasy, making them ideal for daily use, especially in warmer climates or during the daytime.

3. **Gels:** Gel moisturizers have a lightweight, water-based formula that absorbs quickly into the skin, making them suitable for oily or acne-prone skin. They provide hydration without clogging pores, leaving a refreshing, matte finish.

4. **Serums:** Serums are highly concentrated formulations packed with active ingredients like hyaluronic acid, vitamins, and antioxidants. They penetrate deep into the skin, delivering targeted hydration and addressing specific skincare concerns such as fine lines, wrinkles, or hyperpigmentation.

5. **Oils:** Facial oils are rich in fatty acids and antioxidants, providing nourishment and hydration to the skin. They're versatile and can be used alone or mixed with other moisturizers to boost hydration and seal in moisture.

Selecting the right moisturizer involves considering not only your skin type but also any specific concerns or goals you may have, such as anti-aging, acne control, or sensitivity.

Combatting Dryness, Flakiness, and Irritation: Tips for Effective Moisturization

Dryness, flakiness, and irritation are common skincare woes that can be alleviated with proper moisturization. Here are some tips to address these concerns:

1. **Hydrate from Within:** Drink plenty of water to hydrate your skin from the inside out. Aim for at least eight glasses of water per day to maintain optimal hydration levels.

2. **Choose the Right Ingredients:** Look for moisturizers containing hydrating ingredients such as hyaluronic acid, glycerine, ceramides, and niacinamide. These ingredients

help replenish moisture, strengthen the skin barrier, and soothe irritation.

3. **Avoid Harsh Ingredients:** Steer clear of skincare products containing alcohol, fragrance, or sulfates, as these can strip the skin of its natural oils and exacerbate dryness or sensitivity.

4. **Exfoliate Regularly:** Incorporate gentle exfoliation into your skincare routine to remove dead skin cells and promote cell turnover. This helps prevent flakiness and allows moisturizers to penetrate more effectively.

5. **Use Humidifiers:** Invest in a humidifier to add moisture to the air, especially during the dry winter months or in centrally heated or air-conditioned environments. This helps prevent moisture loss from the skin.

6. **Protect Your Skin:** Apply a broad-spectrum sunscreen daily to protect your skin from harmful UV rays, which can further dehydrate the skin and lead to premature aging.

Application Techniques: How Much to Apply and When

Now that you've selected the perfect moisturizer, it's time to master the art of application. Follow these simple techniques for optimal results:

1. **Start with Clean Skin:** Begin with freshly cleansed skin to remove any dirt, oil, or impurities that may hinder moisturizer absorption.

2. **Apply While Skin is Damp:** For maximum hydration, apply moisturizer to slightly damp skin. This helps lock in moisture and ensures better product penetration.

3. **Use Gentle, Upward Strokes:** Gently massage moisturizer into your skin using upward strokes, starting from the center of your face and working outwards. Be sure to cover your entire face, neck, and décolletage.

4. **Don't Forget the Eye Area:** Use a separate eye cream or a pea-sized amount of moisturizer to hydrate the delicate skin around the eyes. Pat gently with your ring finger to avoid tugging or pulling on the skin.

5. **Adjust Quantity Based on Skin Type:** The amount of moisturizer you need varies depending on your skin type. Dry skin may require a larger amount, while oily skin may need only a small dab.

6. **Layering Products:** If using multiple skincare products, apply moisturizer after serums or treatments but before sunscreen during the daytime and after heavier treatments like retinoids or oils at night.

In Conclusion

Moisturization is the cornerstone of a healthy skincare routine, providing essential hydration and nourishment to the skin. By understanding your skin type, selecting the right moisturizer, and adopting effective application techniques, you can achieve a complexion that's hydrated, radiant, and glowing with vitality. So, embrace the power of moisturization and unlock the secret to beautiful, luminous skin.

Chapter 4

Safeguarding Against the Sun: Protecting Your Skin from Harmful UV Rays step 3

One of the most crucial steps in any skincare routine is sun protection. Exposure to the sun's harmful UV rays can lead to premature aging, sunburn, and an increased risk of skin cancer. Therefore, incorporating sunscreen into your daily skincare routine is essential for protecting your skin from sun damage.

When choosing a sunscreen, opt for a broad-spectrum formula that protects against both UVA and UVB rays. Look for a sunscreen with an SPF (sun protection factor) of 30 or higher for adequate protection. Additionally, consider the formulation – whether it's a lotion, gel, or spray – and choose one that feels comfortable on your skin and suits your preferences.

Apply sunscreen generously to all exposed areas of skin, including your face, neck, ears, and any other areas that may be exposed to the sun. Be sure to reapply sunscreen every two hours, or more frequently if you're swimming or sweating heavily.

Shielding Your Skin: The Ultimate Guide to Sun Protection

As the warm rays of the sun beckon us outdoors, it's crucial to remember the importance of protecting our skin from its harmful effects. Sun exposure not only accelerates skin aging but also increases the risk of skin cancer. In this comprehensive guide, we'll explore everything you need to know about sun protection, from choosing the right sunscreen to applying it effectively and understanding the consequences of inadequate protection.

Choosing the Right Sunscreen: Your First Line of Defense

Selecting the right sunscreen is paramount to effective sun protection. Here's what to consider when making your choice:

1. **Broad-Spectrum Protection:** Opt for a sunscreen that offers broad-spectrum protection, meaning it shields against both UVA and UVB rays. UVA rays penetrate deep into the skin, leading to premature aging and increasing the risk of skin cancer, while UVB rays cause sunburn and contribute to skin cancer.

2. **SPF (Sun Protection Factor):** Choose a sunscreen with an SPF of at least 30. SPF indicates how long the sunscreen protects your skin from UVB rays compared to unprotected skin. For example, SPF 30 provides 30 times the protection of bare skin against UVB rays. Higher SPF values offer increased protection, but no sunscreen can provide 100% protection.

3. **Water Resistance:** If you'll be swimming or sweating, opt for a water-resistant sunscreen. Keep in mind that even water-resistant sunscreens require reapplication after swimming or excessive sweating to maintain effectiveness.

4. **Skin Type:** Consider your skin type when selecting a sunscreen. If you have oily or acne-prone skin, choose oil-free or non-comedogenic formulas. For sensitive skin, look for sunscreens labeled as hypoallergenic or fragrance-free.

5. **Additional Features:** Some sunscreens offer additional benefits such as moisturization, antioxidants, or tinted formulations. Choose a sunscreen that aligns with your skincare goals and preferences.

Types of Sunscreen: Understanding the Options

Sunscreen formulations come in various types, each with its unique characteristics and benefits:

1. **Chemical Sunscreens:** Chemical sunscreens work by absorbing UV rays and converting them into heat, which is then released from the skin. They typically contain active ingredients such as avobenzone, octocrylene, or oxybenzone. Chemical sunscreens tend to be lightweight and blend seamlessly into the skin.

2. **Physical (Mineral) Sunscreens:** Physical sunscreens create a physical barrier on the skin's surface, reflecting and scattering UV rays away from the skin. They contain active ingredients like zinc oxide or titanium dioxide. Physical sunscreens are often preferred by those with sensitive skin or allergies to chemical filters, as they are less likely to cause irritation.

3. **Sprays:** Sunscreen sprays offer convenience and ease of application, making them ideal for on-the-go use. However, it's essential to apply sprays generously and evenly to ensure adequate coverage, as it can be challenging to gauge how much product is being dispersed.

4. **Creams and Lotions:** Creams and lotions are traditional sunscreen formulations that provide thorough coverage and hydration. They're suitable for daily use on both the face and body and are available in a wide range of SPF levels and formulations to suit various skin types.

Application Techniques: How to Apply Sunscreen Effectively

Applying sunscreen correctly is crucial for optimal protection against the sun's harmful rays. Follow these steps for effective application:

1. **Apply Generously:** Use a liberal amount of sunscreen to cover all exposed areas of skin thoroughly. The American

Academy of Dermatology recommends applying at least one ounce (about a shot glass full) of sunscreen to cover the entire body.

2. **Don't Forget Often Missed Areas:** Pay special attention to often overlooked areas such as the ears, neck, back of the hands, and tops of the feet. These areas are prone to sunburn but are frequently neglected during sunscreen application.

3. **Reapply Regularly:** Sunscreen should be reapplied every two hours, or more frequently if swimming, sweating, or towel-drying. Remember to reapply immediately after swimming or excessive sweating, even if the sunscreen is labeled as water-resistant.

4. **Apply Before Sun Exposure:** It's essential to apply sunscreen at least 15 minutes before sun exposure to allow the product to absorb into the skin fully. This ensures maximum effectiveness once you're outdoors.

5. **Use in Conjunction with Other Sun Protection Measures:** Sunscreen should be just one component of your sun protection arsenal. Pair it with other protective measures such as seeking shade, wearing protective clothing, and avoiding peak sun hours (10 a.m. to 4 p.m.).

Consequences of Inadequate Sun Protection

Failure to use sunscreen or inadequate protection against the sun's harmful rays can have serious consequences for your skin's health:

1. **Sunburn:** Sunburn is a visible sign of skin damage caused by excessive UV exposure. It can range from mild redness and discomfort to severe pain, blistering, and peeling.

2. **Premature Aging:** Prolonged sun exposure accelerates the aging process, leading to the formation of wrinkles, fine lines, age spots, and a loss of skin elasticity.

3. **Skin Cancer:** UV radiation is a known carcinogen, increasing the risk of developing skin cancer, including melanoma, basal cell carcinoma, and squamous cell carcinoma. Skin cancer is the most common cancer in the United States, with over 5 million cases diagnosed each year.

Reapplication for Ongoing Protection

To maintain continuous protection against the sun's harmful rays, it's essential to reapply sunscreen regularly:

1. **Every Two Hours:** Sunscreen should be reapplied every two hours, even on cloudy days or in the shade. UV rays can penetrate clouds and cause sunburn, so it's crucial to remain vigilant regardless of the weather.

2. **After Swimming or Sweating:** Water-resistant sunscreens provide temporary protection while swimming or sweating, but they still require reapplication every 40 to 80 minutes, depending on the product's water resistance rating.

3. **During Prolonged Sun Exposure:** If you'll be spending an extended period outdoors, consider setting a reminder to reapply sunscreen regularly throughout the day. This ensures continuous protection and reduces the risk of sunburn or skin damage.

In Conclusion

Sun protection is a vital aspect of maintaining healthy, youthful skin and reducing the risk of skin cancer. By choosing the right sunscreen, applying it correctly, and reapplying regularly, you can shield your skin from the sun's harmful rays and enjoy outdoor activities safely. Remember, sun protection is not just a seasonal concern but a year-round necessity for maintaining optimal skin health. So, embrace the power of sun protection and keep your skin radiant, youthful, and protected all year long.

Chapter 5

Addressing Common Skin Concerns: Tailoring Your Skincare Routine

In addition to the basic steps of cleansing, moisturizing, and sun protection, it's important to address any specific skin concerns you may have. Whether it's acne, aging, hyperpigmentation, or sensitivity, there are targeted skincare products and treatments available to help address these issues.

For acne-prone skin, incorporate products containing ingredients such as salicylic acid or benzoyl peroxide to help unclog pores and reduce breakouts. For anti-aging concerns, look for products containing retinoids, vitamin C, or peptides to help stimulate collagen production and reduce the appearance of fine lines and wrinkles.

Hyperpigmentation can be treated with ingredients such as hydroquinone, kojic acid, or niacinamide, which help to inhibit melanin production and lighten dark spots. And for sensitive skin types, opt for gentle, fragrance-free products formulated with soothing ingredients such as aloe vera, chamomile, or oat extract.

Incorporating targeted treatments and products into your skincare routine can help address specific concerns and optimize the health and appearance of your skin.

Nurturing Your Skin for a Lifetime of Radiance

In conclusion, a daily skincare routine is essential for maintaining healthy, radiant skin. By following the steps outlined in this chapter – cleansing, moisturizing, and safeguarding against the sun – you can nurture your skin and protect it from damage. Additionally, by addressing any specific skin concerns you may have, you can tailor your skincare routine to meet your individual needs and achieve your skincare goals. Remember, consistency is key, so make skincare a priority in your daily routine for a lifetime of glowing, youthful skin.

CHAPTER 6

Unlocking Radiant Skin: A Comprehensive Guide to Addressing Common Skin Concerns

In the pursuit of flawless, youthful skin, we often encounter various concerns that can dampen our confidence and hinder our glow. Whether it's acne breakouts, signs of aging, or skin sensitivity, understanding these afflictions and implementing targeted skincare solutions is key to achieving optimal skin health and appearance. In this comprehensive guide, we'll explore common skin concerns, discuss suitable skincare products and treatments, and empower you to take charge of your skin's well-being.

Acne: Banishing Blemishes for Clearer Skin

Acne, characterized by pimples, blackheads, and whiteheads, can wreak havoc on our complexion and self-esteem. But fear not, as there are numerous skincare products and treatments available to combat acne effectively.

1. **Cleansers:** Opt for gentle, non-comedogenic cleansers that remove excess oil and impurities without stripping the skin. Look for ingredients like salicylic acid, benzoyl peroxide, or tea tree oil, known for their acne-fighting properties.

2. **Exfoliants:** Incorporate chemical exfoliants like alpha hydroxy acids (AHAs) or beta hydroxy acids (BHAs) into your skincare routine to unclog pores and remove dead skin cells, preventing acne breakouts. Start with a lower concentration and gradually increase as tolerated.

3. **Spot Treatments:** Target stubborn blemishes with spot treatments containing ingredients like benzoyl peroxide, sulphur, or retinoids. These ingredients help reduce inflammation and accelerate the healing process, minimizing the appearance of acne.

4. **Moisturizers:** Even acne-prone skin requires hydration. Choose oil-free, non-comedogenic moisturizers to prevent clogged pores while keeping the skin hydrated and balanced.

5. **Professional Treatments:** Consider seeking professional treatments such as chemical peels, microdermabrasion, or laser therapy to address persistent acne or acne scarring. Consult with a dermatologist to determine the best course of action for your skin.

Aging: Embracing Youthful Skin at Any Age

As we age, our skin undergoes various changes, including the formation of fine lines, wrinkles, and sagging. However, with the right skincare regimen and targeted treatments, we can defy the signs of aging and maintain a youthful complexion.

1. **Retinoids:** Incorporate retinoids, derivatives of vitamin A, into your skincare routine to stimulate collagen production, reduce fine lines, and improve skin texture. Start with a lower strength and gradually increase as tolerated to minimize irritation.

2. **Antioxidants:** Look for skincare products containing antioxidants like vitamin C, vitamin E, and green tea extract to neutralize free radicals, prevent oxidative stress, and protect the skin from environmental damage. These ingredients also promote collagen synthesis and brighten the complexion.

3. **Peptides:** Peptides are amino acids that help boost collagen production, improve skin elasticity, and reduce the appearance of wrinkles. Incorporate peptide-rich serums or creams into your skincare routine for firmer, more youthful-looking skin.

4. **Hydration:** Hydrated skin appears plumper and more youthful. Use moisturizers containing hyaluronic acid, glycerin, or ceramides to lock in moisture and restore the skin's natural barrier function.

5. **Sun Protection:** Sun exposure accelerates skin aging, leading to wrinkles, age spots, and sagging. Apply a broad-spectrum sunscreen with SPF 30 or higher daily to protect your skin from harmful UV rays and prevent premature aging.

Sensitive Skin: Nurturing Delicate Complexions with Care

Sensitive skin is prone to redness, irritation, and inflammation, often triggered by environmental factors, skincare products, or underlying conditions. Gentle, soothing skincare products and treatments are essential for managing sensitive skin effectively.

1. **Hypoallergenic Formulations:** Choose skincare products labeled as hypoallergenic, fragrance-free, and non-irritating to minimize the risk of sensitivity reactions. Look for soothing ingredients like chamomile, aloe vera, and oat extract to calm and nourish sensitive skin.

2. **Minimalist Skincare Routine:** Simplify your skincare routine by using a minimal number of products to reduce the risk of irritation. Focus on gentle cleansers, hydrating moisturizers, and sunscreen formulated for sensitive skin.

3. **Patch Testing:** Before trying a new skincare product, perform a patch test on a small area of skin to assess for

any adverse reactions. Apply a small amount of product to the inner forearm or behind the ear and monitor for redness, itching, or irritation.

4. **Avoid Harsh Ingredients:** Steer clear of skincare products containing harsh ingredients such as alcohol, fragrances, sulfates, and artificial dyes, as these can exacerbate sensitivity and inflammation.

5. **Consult with a Dermatologist:** If you struggle with persistent sensitivity or skin conditions like rosacea or eczema, consult with a dermatologist for personalized skincare recommendations and treatment options tailored to your specific needs.

Optimizing Skin Health and Appearance: A Holistic Approach

Addressing specific skin concerns not only improves the appearance of your complexion but also enhances overall skin health and vitality. By incorporating targeted skincare products and treatments into your daily routine, you can achieve a radiant, youthful complexion and feel confident in your skin at any age.

Remember, consistency is key when it comes to skincare. Stick to your regimen, be patient with your skin, and don't hesitate to seek professional advice if needed. With dedication and the right approach, you can unlock the secret to radiant, healthy skin that radiates confidence and beauty from within.

Chapter 7

The Importance of a Long-Term Skin Care Regimen for Appearance and Health

Taking care of your skin is not just about looking good; it's also about maintaining overall health. A long-term skin care regimen can have profound effects on both your appearance and your general well-being. From preventing premature aging to reducing the risk of skin conditions, here's why investing in a daily skin care routine is crucial.

1. Maintaining Youthful Appearance:

A consistent skin care routine can help keep your skin looking youthful and radiant. Cleansing, moisturizing, and protecting your skin from the sun's harmful rays are essential steps in preventing wrinkles, fine lines, and age spots. Incorporating anti-aging ingredients such as retinoids and antioxidants can further boost collagen production and repair damaged skin cells, promoting a smoother and more youthful complexion over time.

2. Preventing Skin Conditions:

Regular cleansing and exfoliation can help prevent clogged pores and breakouts by removing dirt, oil, and dead skin cells that can lead to acne. Additionally, using products with ingredients like salicylic acid or benzoyl peroxide can target acne-causing bacteria and reduce inflammation, keeping breakouts at bay. For those with sensitive skin or conditions like eczema or rosacea, a gentle and hydrating skincare routine can help soothe irritation and minimize flare-ups.

3. Protecting Against Environmental Damage:

Exposure to environmental pollutants and UV radiation can accelerate skin aging and increase the risk of skin cancer. Incorporating sunscreen with broad-spectrum protection into your daily routine can shield your skin from harmful UV rays and prevent sunburns, hyperpigmentation, and skin cancer. Antioxidants like vitamin C and E can also help neutralize free radicals caused by environmental stressors, further protecting your skin from damage.

4. Boosting Confidence and Mental Well-being:

Taking care of your skin can also have psychological benefits, boosting your confidence and self-esteem. When you feel good about your appearance, you're more likely to project positivity and confidence in your personal and professional life. Additionally, the act of self-care involved in a skincare routine can be a form of stress relief and relaxation, promoting overall mental well-being.

Consequences of Neglecting a Skin Care Routine:

Failing to adhere to a daily skin care routine can have detrimental effects on both your skin's appearance and health. Without proper cleansing and moisturizing, dirt, oil, and bacteria can accumulate on the skin's surface, leading to clogged pores, breakouts, and dullness. Skipping sunscreen can leave your skin vulnerable to sun damage, including sunburns, premature aging, and an increased risk of skin cancer.

Moreover, neglecting skincare can exacerbate existing skin conditions like acne, eczema, and rosacea, causing discomfort and potentially worsening symptoms over time. Without adequate protection and nourishment, the skin's natural barrier function may weaken, making it more susceptible to environmental stressors and infections.

Conclusion:

A long-term skin care regimen is essential for maintaining both the appearance and health of your skin. By investing in a daily routine that includes cleansing, moisturizing, sun protection, and targeted treatments, you can achieve a radiant complexion while safeguarding against premature aging and skin conditions. Remember, consistency is key, so make skincare a priority in your daily routine for long-lasting benefits.